# Known Cancer Cures

## Cancer Cures Revisited

Ryder Management Inc.

ISBN: **1505248167**
ISBN-13: **978-1505248166**

# Epigraph

*"First, do no harm."*
*Hippocrates - the Father of Medicine.*

.

# Table of Contents

# Introduction

Being told that you have cancer has to be one of the darkest moments anyone can ever experience. Your Oncologist or Cancer Doctor will then insist on your instant acceptance of one or more of the traditional cancer treatments being "surgery, chemotherapy or radiation", otherwise known as "cut, poison or burn". One is faced with an endless stream of medical tests, examinations, medications, follow-up tests, new tests, new drugs, support therapy and opinions, all while you are plunged into an abyss that will dramatically change your life forever.

In the early 1900' s, one in twenty people were diagnosed with cancer; in the 1940 's, one in sixty people had cancer; in the 1970' s this ratio was one out of every ten people and today, the number of people diagnosed with cancer is one out of every two people.

Cancer is big business. It is estimated that the cancer industry today is worth well over $ 125 billion dollars.

With all the money being raised for cancer research, why has the industry not found a cure? The fact is, there has always been a cure for cancer, even multiple cures, but the pharmaceutical industry is more concerned with profits and not patients.

The purpose of this book is not to disclose the lies of conventional medicine; rather, the purpose of this book is enlightenment. The intention of this book is to provide you with facts on real cures for cancer. I know cancer can be cured because I killed my own cancer.

Reference and citations to many other people's studies have also been included in order to provide you with additional sources of research and further reading.

The goal of this book is to provide you with hope, not despair, as you decide on how you will treat your cancer. It is a compilation of sorts, of what helped me cure my cancer.

# FDA on Cancer

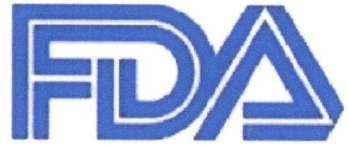

The Food and Drug Administration (the FDA) is a not for profit organization and accordingly, is ran by an elected board of directors. Since its inception however, the various senior members of the FDA rotate lucrative positions on the boards of major drug companies and other key organizations. It has been found that the FDA has very serious and severe conflicts of interest, including owning stocks in the very corporations they are supposed to be "monitoring, policing and controlling".

Included on the FDA's website under "What We Do", you will find the following:

"FDA is responsible for protecting the public health by assuring the safety, efficacy and security of human and veterinary drugs, biological products, medical devices, our nation's food supply, cosmetics, and products that emit radiation."

*http:// www.fda.gov/ AboutFDA/ Transparency/ Basics/ ucm194879. Htm*

The majority of the funding received by the FDA is from the pharmaceutical industry. Also noteworthy and important to keep in mind, "Quackery" is synonymous to "competition".

A highly educational documentary that is available on YouTube by Massimo Mazzucco entitled "Cancer: The Forbidden Cures" is described by Dr. Mercola as follows:

*"A fascinating documentary that exposes the corruption of the cancer industry and the extreme measures they will undertake to discredit, imprison, and professionally destroy any physician who treats cancer patients naturally"*

It should also be noted that it is necessary to be apprised of the source of your research. Companies that are in bed with Big Pharma will not provide you with facts that are to your benefit. Examples include PubMed, Wikipedia, etc.

The following pages discuss various proven cancer cures: Cures that the FDA and conventional medicine have gone to great lengths to discredit.

# Known Cancer Cures

Food Grade Hydrogen Peroxide (H202)

Cannabis Oil (a.k.a. Rick Simpson Oil)

Turmeric (curcumin)

Essiac Tea

Graviola or Soursop

Mistletoe

Vitamin B17 (laetrile)

DMSO

Vitamin D

Dr. Max Gerson

Dr. Burzynski

Royal Raymond Rife

Dr. Hulda Clark

Harry Hoxsey

# Food Grade Hydrogen Peroxide (H202)

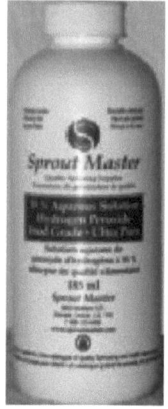

Nobel Prize winner, Dr. Otto Heinrich Warburg devoted his life to studying the causes of cancer. In his paper published on March 7, 1927 entitled "The Metabolism of Tumors in the Body", Dr. Warburg wrote, "All normal cells have an absolute requirement for oxygen, but cancer cells can live without oxygen - a rule without exception. Deprive a cell 35% of its oxygen for 48 hours and it may become cancerous."

His paper began by stating the assumption that "tumor cells obtain the energy required for their existence in two ways: by respiration and by fermentation." Dr. Warburg made the connection that lack of oxygen (or hypoxia) and acidosis are "two sides of the same coin - where there is one, there is the other." He went on to state:

*"Cancerous tissue is acidic, whereas healthy tissue is alkaline. Water splits into H + and OH- ions, if there is an excess of H +, it is acidic; if there is an excess of OH- ions, then it is alkaline."*

For complete, in-depth information on using Food Grade Hydrogen Peroxide, this author recommends the Kindle eBook, by Sharon Daniels entitled, "Hydrogen Peroxide Miracle Healers from the Kitchen". Her research reveals that "as far back as the early 19th century, doctors used H2O2 therapy to treat bacterial infections, including syphilis, which were infections resistant to other forms of treatment. In the beginning of the 20th century, medical doctors used H2O2 therapy to treat bacterial infections, including syphilis, which were infections resistant to other forms of treatment. In the beginning of the 20th century, medical doctors used H2O2 therapy to treat a wide array of diseases including asthma, whooping cough, ulcers, tuberculosis and typhoid fever.

However, for reasons that remain unclear today, the success of H2O2 treatment was ignored by many medical professionals and instead, high priced pharmaceuticals were prescribed to patients to treat the same diseases that H2O2 cures."

# Cannabis Oil (a.k.a. Rick Simpson Oil or RSO)

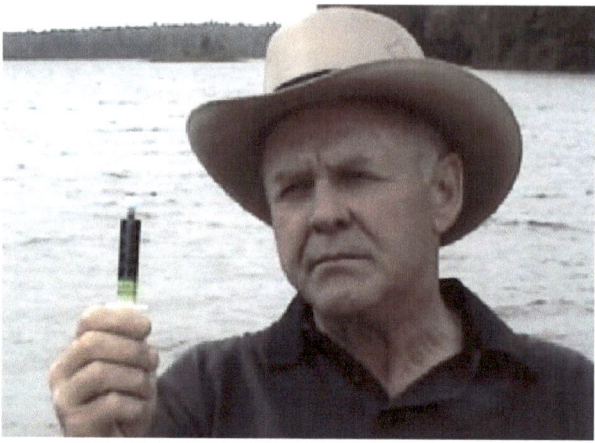

I was apprised and subsequently insisted upon using "Rick Simpson Oil (RSO)". What this means is that it is cannabis or hash oil that is a known cancer cure. I choose to refer to this oil as "Rick Simpson Oil" as that is who has selflessly travelled the world for the purpose of informing, educating and ultimately saving people's lives. I know he saved my life by informing me on the true value in the cannabis plant.

Cannabis is unique in that it produces phyto-cannabinoids, and when these phyto-cannabinoids meet up with our body's endocannabinoid system, it has been said that it is a marriage made in heaven due to the synergy effect.

To gain a preliminary understanding of Cannabinoids and Terpenes, please see our book "Cannabinoids and Terpenes The Medicinal Benefits of Cannabis" available at Amazon.

It is very unfortunate that this plant was removed from the Pharmacopeia for the purpose of allowing Big Pharma to rise.

To learn how to make this medicine, please review the information contained at "Cure Your Own Cancer" or "Phoenix Tears".

# Turmeric (Curcumin)

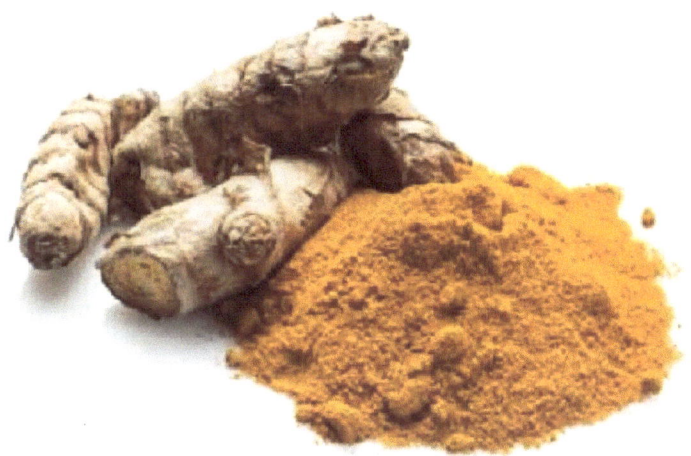

In December 1993, the University of Mississippi Medical Center filed for a patent on turmeric and in March 1995 they were granted US patent #5401504 using turmeric as a wound healing agent. However, in 1996, the Indian Council of Scientific and Industrial Research challenged the patent on the grounds that it was not new nor novel.

This wasn't the first time that the Western World claimed inventions, which were known to India for centuries as their own.

Although conventional medicine may try to mock turmeric as a cancer cure, a 2014 study on turmeric, published in "Cancer Letters" entitled "Targeting Cancer Stem Cells by Curcumin and Clinical Applications" (PMID 24463298) has demonstrated the anticancer effect of curcumin on cancer cells. Curcumin is the polyphenol derived from the rhizomes of turmeric, the Indian spice. Turmeric is also related to ginger.

To get the full benefits of curcumin, it is important to understand that turmeric is very poorly absorbed in our body. The reason for this is that turmeric is fat-soluble, meaning that it must be dissolved in fat in order to reach your blood, where it can offer its greatest benefits. In addition, using peppercorn with turmeric can increase its effectiveness by 1,000 times.

Please see Ryder Management Inc.'s book on Turmeric entitled *"Turmeric: A Cancer Cure The Amazing Health and Beauty Benefits of Turmeric"* for more in-depth information on turmeric. This book is available at Amazon.

# Essiac Tea

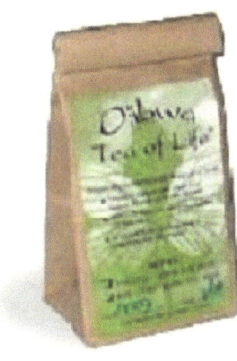

The ingredients that are used in Essiac Tea were selflessly provided by Ojibwa First People early in the last century. The herbs that make up this concoction include the following:

Burdock Root 54%: increases circulation; destroys bacteria and fungus, anti-tumor, reduces cell mutation;

Sheep Sorrel 35%: rich in Vitamin A, B, C, D, K and E; also includes calcium, iron, magnesium, silicon, zinc, manganese, iodine and copper;

Slippery Elm Bark 9%: relieves inflammatory symptoms, anti-biotic, antimicrobial, and is able to remove toxins;

Turkey Rhubarb Root 2%: used in TCM for its detoxifying properties in the liver, antibiotic, anti-microbial, anti-tumor

From the website www.ojibwatea.com, the following history on Essiac Tea can be found:

*"In the mid-1920s, Rene Caisse was head nurse at the Sisters of Providence Hospital in a northern Ontario town. While on duty, Rene was bathing an elderly lady and noticed that one of her breasts had a lot of scar tissue on it. Upon questioning the lady, she learned that the women had advanced breast cancer 30 years earlier. The woman further explained that she had met an old Indian medicine man who told her he could cure her cancer. She said that she had no money at that time, and didn't want to have an operation anyway, so she went to see the Indian. He showed her certain herbs growing in the area and told her to pick them and make a tea and to drink it every day.*

*She had no reoccurrence of cancer to that day, 30 years later.*

*In 1922, Rene named the formula "Essiac" after the backward spelling of her own last name, Caisse. The recipe from "a very old Indian Medicine Man," allows for many stories and theories. There has never been "proof" of the actual tribal heritage of the Medicine Man who offered this formula, as many Native American Tribes lived in the area at the time.*

*Rene Caisse spent her life working with this herb tea, until she died in 1978 at the age of 90. For a time, the Canadian Minister of Health allowed Rene to treat certain terminally ill patients in her Bracebridge clinic. According to Rene, many of the people she treated reported they were helped by the remedy while others claimed living with their illness was made more bearable."*

# Graviola or Soursop

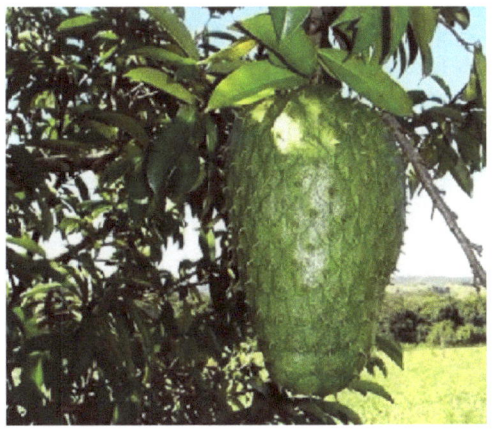

Graviola or Soursop, as it is known in South America, is an extremely important and sacred gift from the heavens. In South America, where it is also known as guanabana, the fruit, bark, roots, leaves and seeds of the Graviola tree all have a purpose in traditional healing. The seeds and fruit obtained from this tree are an effective remedy in eradicating worms, lice and other parasites.

Since the 1940's, scientific research has been carried out on the active ingredients and compounds found in Soursop and their effect on cancer. A study released in 1998 shows the chemical compounds and particularly acetogennis, perform anti-cancerous , anti-tumorous and anti-viral activities.

Studies reveal that Soursop leaves are effective in eliminating all forms of cancer. The say that money does not grow on trees, but the cure for cancer does.

Soursop grows from the Graviola tree and can be found in countries such as Mexico, Central America, South America, Cuba and Caribbean Islands. The tree can reach heights of 30 feet and the Soursop fruit can grow to 12 inches in length and weigh over six pounds.

# Mistletoe

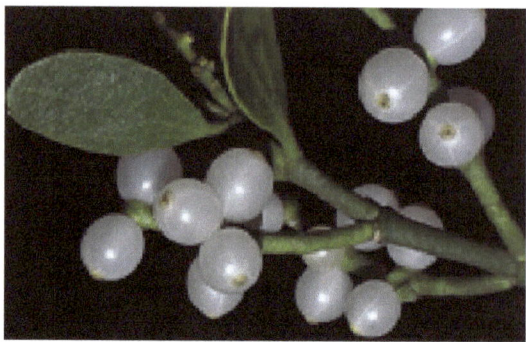

Mistletoe is what Suzanne Sumers used to treat her breast cancer.

Studies show that mistletoe greatly increases the immune factors in our body, It was widely regarded as a relatively cure-all by ancient Greeks. As a cancer cure, mistletoe extracts are already authorized for use in Europe as a treatment for colon cancer and various other forms of cancer including rectal, stomach and breast cancers. Unfortunately, the FDA does not authorize mistletoe for use in the United States.

Mistletoe is a semi parasitic plant that receives its nourishment by growing on various trees including apple, birch, elm, maple, oak and pine. Mistletoe contains chlorophyll and is capable of undergoing photosynthesis and has been found to be an effective treatment for arthritis, epilepsy, hypertension, menopause, in addition to cancer.

Laboratory studies have shown that mistletoe extracts, known as iscador, are found to be proapoptotic toward cancer cells, meaning that they promote cell death. This is not new information as it has been used for over one hundred years as a cancer treatment.

# Vitamin B17 and Laetrile

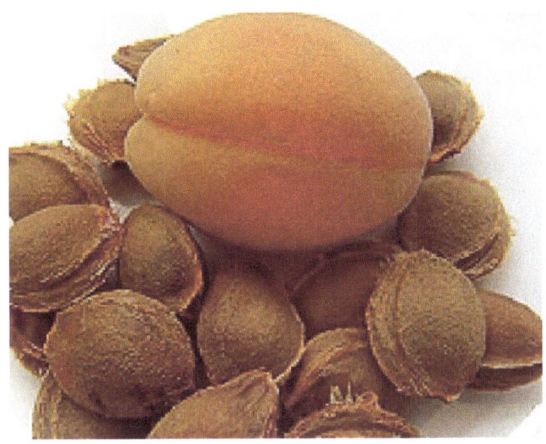

Laetrile (Vitamin B17 or amygdalin) therapy is one of the most popular and best known natural cancer treatments in the Western world. Laetrile works by targeting and killing cancer cells at the same time that it builds the immune system. However, laetrile was banned by the FDA in 1971 despite its proven efficacy. In fact, many people still falsely believe, thanks to the FDA, that amygdalin (or laetrile or B17) poses a serious cyanide poisoning and therefore, toxic threat. This is a false flag.

The best source of amygdalin or laetrile is found in the apricot seed (or kernel).

Paul Reid, a 68 year old Australian, went public after curing his incurable lymphoma thirteen years ago by consuming 30 apricot kernels per day.

While using any form of cancer treatment, it is important to also be on an organic diet, eliminating and avoiding all processed foods.

For additional information on Vitamin B17, please see the book "World Without Cancer: The Story of Vitamin B17" by G. Edward Griffin.

# DMSO

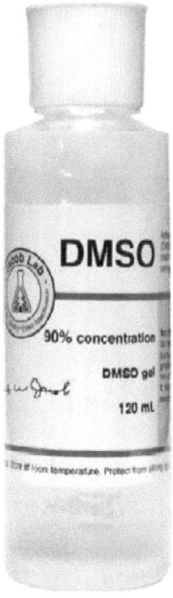

DMSO or dimethyl sulfoxide was discovered by Russian scientist Alexander Zaytsev in 1866 as a by-product of wood pulp processing. It was subsequently discovered that DMSO was an effective cancer treatment as it targeted cancer cells without causing damage to healthy cells. DMSO became known as the "Magic Bullet for Cancer".

James L. Goddard, known as the crusading FDA leader during the 1960's, was also responsible for his persecution of DMSO, a simple molecule that also provided miraculous pain relief and offered unprecedented advancements for the medical community, including cancer.

The FDA has never admitted to its errors regarding their quashing of DMSO although the positive studies from qualified scientists amount to well over a thousand. At the same time, the FDA's criticisms over DSMO have been shown to be almost totally based on lies or unsubstantiated rumors. Even twenty years later, in the late 1980s, the FDA continued to imprison DMSO advocates.

"The malignity of Goddard's arbitrary and conscienceless acts in 1966-1968 against reputable scientists, dedicated doctors and the public good is one of the darkest chapters of FDA history." (www.sntp.net)

However, in addition to the FDA's crusade against DMSO, a number of pharmaceutical companies continue to suppress what some call "the major drug of the century" fearing that their individual profits were at stake. Dr. Charles c. Edwards, the then Commissioner of the FDA, testified before congress by stating, "It is not the FDA's policy to jeopardize the financial interests of the pharmaceutical companies".

Dr. Jacob, who, in 1961, was head of the organ transplant program at Oregon Health Sciences University, summarized that the reason DMSO, a natural healer, was left on the sidelines is because "it doesn't follow the rifle approach of one agent against one disease entity."

In addition to effectively treating cancer, DMSDO is also an effective pain reliever; reduces inflammation, is able to soften collagen in scleroderma; eases arthritis; along with having so much more potential.

Dr. Jacob continues to believe that DMSO should not even be called a drug but is more correctly a new therapeutic principle, with an effect on medicine that will be profound in many areas.

See also:

*"DMSO: Nature's Healer" by Morton Walker;*

*"DMSO: Many Uses, Much Controversy" by Maya Muir*

# Vitamin D

| Age group | Recommended Dietary Allowance (RDA) per day | Tolerable Upper Intake Level (UL) per day |
|---|---|---|
| Infants 0-6 months | 400 IU (10 mcg) * | 1000 IU (25 mcg) |
| Infants 7-12 months | 400 IU (10 mcg) * | 1500 IU (38 mcg) |
| Children 1-3 years | 600 IU (15 mcg) | 2500 IU (63 mcg) |
| Children 4-8 years | 600 IU (15 mcg) | 3000 IU (75 mcg) |
| Children and Adults 9-70 years | 600 IU (15 mcg) | 4000 IU (100 mcg) |
| Adults > 70 years | 800 IU (20 mcg) | 4000 IU (100 mcg) |
| Pregnancy & Lactation | 600 IU (15 mcg) | 4000 IU (100 mcg) |

*Adequate Intake rather than Recommended Dietary Allowance

Dr. Mercola describes Vitamin D as "a steroid hormone that is capable of influencing almost every cell in the human body, making it one of nature's most potent cancer fighters. Receptors in the human body that responds to Vitamin D have been found in nearly every type of human cell, from your bones to your brain." (www.mercola.com).

Anytime research was publicized on the importance of increasing Vitamin D intake, the advice from the media that accompanied the research would include a paragraph that stated "current recommended daily allowance from the Institute of Medicine calls for 200 IU/ day from birth through age 50 years and 400 IU/ day thereafter. "

However, Vitamin D deficiency continues to rise. Why? The answer is because 200 IU per day is far too low. In addition, we have come to falsely believe that unless we apply a strong sunscreen when in the sun, we are at greater risk for cancer. This too is far from the truth. Strict sun protection has been shown to exacerbate Vitamin D deficiency.

Diseases that are prevented by Vitamin D include: Cancer of all types; high blood pressure , osteoporosis; rickets; depression; diabetes; heart disease; kidney disease; tuberculosis; influenza; hair loss, dementia including Alzheimer's and more.

Chemical compounds found in SPF sunscreen lotions are mostly synthetic and have a highly toxic effect on and in the human body. Coconut oil is a natural and safe alternative to cancer causing commercial sunscreens.

In his book, "the Coconut Oil Miracle", Dr. Bruce Fife says, *"The first commercial suntan and sun screen lotions contained coconut oil as their primary ingredient. Even today many sun screen lotions include coconut oil in their formulas. Coconut oil has an amazing ability to heal the skin and block the damaging effects of UV radiation from the sun. One of the reasons why it is so effective in protecting the skin is its antioxidant properties, which helps prevent burning and oxidative damage that promotes skin cancer."*

# Dr. Max Gerson

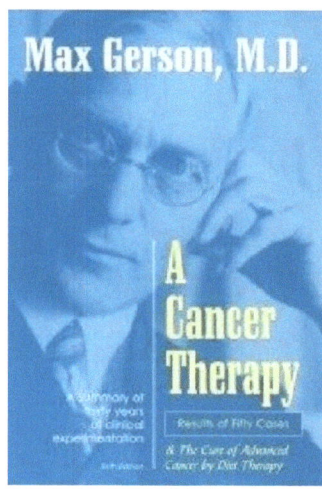

"Dr. Gerson's daughter, Charlotte Gerson, founded the Gerson Institute in 1977, "to spread awareness of the Gerson Therapy and make it available to people across the world. The Gerson Institute is the true source of information on the original, proven Gerson Therapy.

The Gerson Therapy is a safe, natural treatment developed by Dr. Max Gerson in the 1920s. The Therapy activates the body's extraordinary ability to heal itself through an organic, vegetarian diet, raw juices, coffee enemas and natural supplements. The Gerson Therapy treats the underlying causes of disease: toxicity and nutritional deficiency.

The Gerson Therapy is a non-specific treatment that effectively treats many different conditions by healing the body as a whole, rather than selectively targeting a specific condition or symptom. Over the past 60 years, thousands of people have used the Gerson Therapy to recover from so-called "incurable" diseases, including: Cancer, Diabetes, Heart Disease, Arthritis, Auto-immune disorders, and so much more".

www.gerson.org

Thank you Charlotte Gerson!

# Royal Raymond Rife

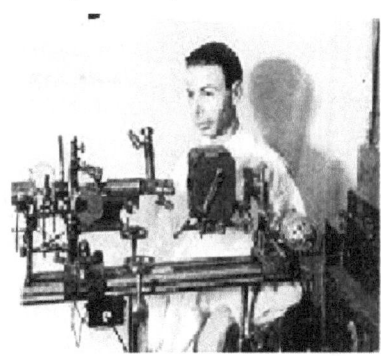

Similar to Dr. Max Gerson and others, Roy Rife also met with massive resistance from the orthodox medical industry in his pursuit of making a cancer cure available to the masses. The following is an excerpt from the book "The Cancer Cure that Worked" by Barry Lynes:

"Royal R. Rife, born in 1888, was one of the greatest scientific geniuses of the 20th century. He began researching a cure for cancer in 1920, and by 1932 he had isolated the cancer virus. He learned how to destroy it in laboratory cultures and went on to cure cancer in animals. In 1934, he opened a clinic which successfully cured 16 of 16 cases within three months' time. Working with some of the most respected researchers in America along with leading doctors from Southern California, he electronically destroyed the cancer virus in patients, allowing their own immune systems to restore health. A special Research Committee of the University of Southern California oversaw the laboratory research and the experimental treatments until the end of the 1930' s. Follow-up clinics conducted in 1935, 1936, and 1937 by the head of the U.S.C. Medical Committee verified the results of the 1934 clinic. Independent physicians utilizing the equipment successfully treated as many as 40 people per day during these years. In addition to curing cancer and other deadly diseases, degenerative conditions such as cataracts were reversed. Rife had been able to determine the precise electrical frequency which destroyed individual microorganisms responsible for cancer, herpes, tuberculosis, and other illnesses. His work was described in Science magazine, medical journals, and later the Smithsonian Institution's annual report.

Unfortunately, Rife's scientific theories and methods of treatment conflicted with orthodox views. His work was stopped and both the research and the treatments were forced underground."

Today, most Naturopathic Doctors utilize the Rife machine where it is known as "electromagnetic therapy". The machine is very effective but unfortunately the FDA, Cancer.org and many other organizations are still on the warpath to discredit this invention.

# Dr. Burzynski

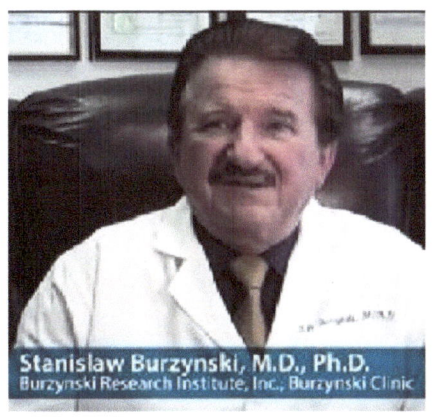

Stanislaw Burzynski, M.D., Ph.D.
Burzynski Research Institute, Inc., Burzynski Clinic

After the Italian fashion model Fabio Lanzoni exhausted all sources of conventional medicine in an effort to save his sister from the wrath of ovarian cancer, Fabio turned to the Burzynski Clinic. In an interview, Fabio, referring to Dr. Burzynski states, "He is a genius. He definitely, I believe, he has the cure for cancer… They have to let him get his office back and let him do his work…"

The long continuing saga and court battle regarding the Food & Drug Administration vs. Stanislaw Burzynski, MD, PhD, is mind boggling. Dr. Burzynski did however; win the largest and possibly most convoluted legal struggle against the Food and Drug Administration in US history. The court battle and struggle was about his patented cancer treatment and how it threatened the entire paradigm of the money making industry being that of the cancer industry.

# Dr. Hulda Clark

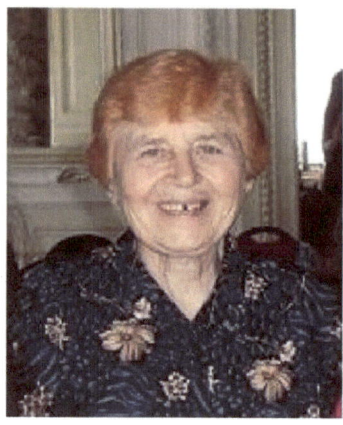

Dr. Hulda Clark (1928 - 2009) believed that cancer is caused by a parasitic infection that can be cured with an herbal mixture. In her most recent book, The Cure for All Diseases, she describes an electronic device called a zapper that can also cure cancer, along with a host of other diseases.

Many Homeopaths and Naturopaths also agree that most cancers begin with a parasitic infection. It is interesting to note the correlation between Dr. Clark's work and that of Rene Caisse and Dr. Max Gerson as all four therapies involve ridding the body of toxins and parasites and then subsequently nourishing the body and treating it for vitamin deficiency.

There are hundreds of people who have given testimony of the success of the herbal treatment by Dr. Clark where they have completely stopped the progress of cancer in their bodies with herbal treatment that include anti-parasitic herbs.

The herbs, along with their description, are:

BLACK WALNUT HULLS (from the black walnut tree or juglans nigra)

Used by North American Natives as an anti-parasitic, anti-bacterial, antiviral and antifungal remedy, the active ingredients are juglone, tannin and iodine. The tincture of the green hulls of black walnut kills parasites in their adult stage.

WORMWOOD (from the Artemisia shrub or artemisia absinthum)

Known for its vermicidal properties, wormwood helps those with a weak and under-active digestive system. It increases the acidity of the stomach and the production of bile. Wormwood capsules are also known to kill the larval stage of parasites

COMMON CLOVES (from the clove tree or Eugenia caryophyllata)

Anti-parasitic, anti-fungal, antiviral and anti-inflammatory properties, common cloves also have the ability as an effective pain relief and clove capsules are also used to remove the eggs of parasites.

# Harry Hoxsey

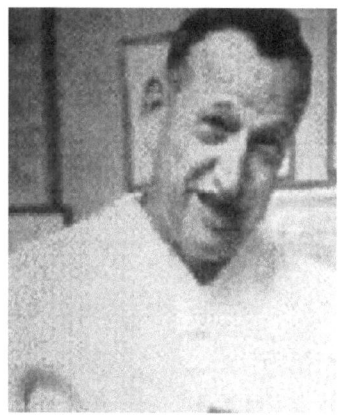

Harry Hoxsey (1902 – 1974) obtained his family's secret anti-cancer recipe from his father, when his father was on his death bed and spent the majority of his life fighting to save lives from the wrath of conventional cancer therapy. The Hoxsey family anti-cancer recipe consisted of the following herbs:

Burdock root: antibacterial, antifungal, blood purifier, prevents liver damage, among other beneficial qualities.

Red Clover Blossom;

Licorice Root;

Buckthorn Aged Bark;

Stillingia Root;

Poke Root;

Barberry Root Bark;

Oregon grape Root;

Wild Indigo Root;

Prickly Ash Bark;

Kelp.

# Conclusion

The purpose of this book was that of information, education and to assure you that you are not alone, that there is hope and that you do have a choice when it comes to your medical decisions. Please take a step back and think about the information presented with an objective and logical frame of mind.

My hope with publishing this book is to save more people from the wrath of conventional cancer treatment.

In the last hundred years, man has advanced as a result of many discoveries. However, we are told that we have the knowledge of putting a man on the moon, but why is it that we are lead to believe that a cure for cancer has not been found? The truth is, there has always been a cure for cancer, in fact, there are many cures, and all you need to do is to choose an effective one; one that will not harm you.

Conventional medicine is also referred to as "Orthodox Medicine". Orthodox is defined as "conforming to established or accepted standards" and "conforming to the Christian faith as established by the early Church".

# Other Sources of Reference and Assistance

## Websites:

Truly Organic Foods: http://www.trulyorganicfoods.com/

Cancer Tutor: www.cancertutor.com

Cure Your Own Cancer:  www.cureyourowncancer.org

Ryder Management Inc:  http://rydermanagement.ca

Natural Health News: www.naturalnews.com

Dr. Mercola: www.mercola.com

The Gerson Therapy: www.gerson.org

Ojibwa Tea Life: www.ojibwatea.com

The Cancer Racket Begins by Wade Frazer:

http://www.ahealedplanet.net/medicine.htm

## Books:

*Hydrogen Peroxide Cures* by Sharon Daniels

*Cancer: Amazing Cures for Cancer You Need to Know Now* by Ryan Seager

*A Cancer Cure? The Amazing Health and Beauty Benefits of Turmeric* by Ryder Management Inc.

*Cannabinoids and Terpenes The Medicinal Benefits of Cannabis* by Ryder Management Inc.

*World Without Cancer: The Story of Vitamin B17* by G. Edward Griffin.

# Closing Remarks

*"It's painful not to be treated as an equal. You have to be strong to walk through the storm. It's like being a bridge between two worlds. If this is the case, all I ask is for people to wash their feet before they try to walk on me."*
*Alanis Obomsawin*

*"Christopher Columbus is a symbol, not of a man, but of imperialism. Imperialism and colonialism are not something that happened decades ago or generations ago, but they are still happening now with the exploitation of people."*
*John Mohawk*

# About the Author

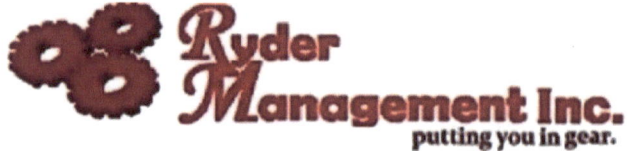

Ryder Management Inc. (Rydermgt or RMI) is a Canadian Controlled Private Corporation (CCPC) based in London, ON Canada. As an "umbrella" organization, RMI brings together a group of authors whom are professionals in their respective fields and are writing with the primary goal of providing books that educate, comfort and offer assurance that natural remedies do exist and are an effective and safe way to enhance health.

The contributing author of our first book "*A Cancer Cure? The Amazing Health and Beauty Benefits of Turmeric*" was diagnosed with cancer and adamantly refused conventional cancer treatment used in Canada. Stephanie then began a quest for an alternative method of treatment that included online research, interviews and placing calls to India. This first book begins the series on herbal remedies that date back to ancient times!